Intimacy

Nurturing Deeper Connections in Relationships

By: Somtoochukwu Justin

Copyright

Table if contents

Listen to the story of this two Lovers (Alex and Olivia)

Once upon a time in the charming town of Evergreen, two people were destined for an extraordinary journey of love and closeness. Alex and Olivia were two lovers whose story was like a tapestry made of threads of enthusiasm, vulnerability, and the promise to uncover the profundities of their bond.

Their story started with a fortunate experience at a nearby book shop. Alex, an aspiring artist with a talent for sketching, was captivated by Olivia's chuckling as she looked through the pages of a novel. When their eyes met, it seemed like the universe was conspiring to bring these two kindred spirits together.

As they moved into the beginning phases of their relationship, Alex and Olivia found the delight of shared encounters. From sudden picnics in the park to late-night talks under a sky loaded with stars, they found comfort in one another's presence. Their relationship deepened with each shared mystery, each vulnerable disclosure.

Intimacy was like a fragile move between vulnerability and trust. Alex, somewhat reluctant to express his feelings, found the intensity of opening up to Olivia. Gradually, he uncovered the layers of his past, fears, and dreams, finding solace in Olivia's unyielding acknowledgment and comprehension.

Their love experienced its offer of tempests. Outer weights, misjudgments, and the heaviness of duties attempted to make breaks in their association. Be that as it may, Alex and Olivia weathered these difficulties together, understanding that the intensity of their bond was in their capacity to explore difficulty hand in hand.

As people, Alex and Olivia started on trips of individual development. They bolstered one another's aspirations and dreams, perceiving that individual satisfaction was fundamental to the flourishing of their shared connection. In commending one another's successes, they found that development was not a danger yet a remunerating power inside their relationship.

The physical measurement of their love unfurled with delicacy and energy. Intimacy for Alex and Olivia was not just a physical demonstration yet a language of association—expressing wants, advancing closeness, and finding the subtleties of joy that brought them nearer with each touch.

As time advanced, Alex and Olivia praised achievements. Anniversaries denoted not just the progression of time yet the deepening of their promise. They made customs, from cutting their initials on a preferred tree to returning to the book shop where their eyes initially met, weaving a story of shared encounters that turned into the establishment of their closeness.

In the present day, Alex and Olivia's romantic tale keeps on unfurling. Their excursion with intimacy is continuous, a continuous investigation of the intricate strings that tie them together. They've realized that intimacy is not a goal yet a journey—a journey they've grasped with open hearts, a readiness to develop, and an unyielding promise to uncover the excellence of their bond.

As Alex and Olivia explore the tapestry of their love, they convey with them the exercises learned, the delights shared, and the expectation of the sections yet to be composed—a romantic tale that stands as a declaration to the enduring intensity of intimacy in the move of two spirits intertwined.

Introduction:

Welcome to " Intimacy: Nurturing Deeper Connections in Relationships," a journey into the depths of human connection. In a world of constant change and evolving dynamics, the pursuit of lasting and fulfilling connections has become a universal desire. As we explore the complexities of modern relationships, the need to foster intimacy—authentic, deep, and transformative—becomes increasingly important.

This book is not a roadmap to a utopian ideal, but a compass for those navigating the ever-changing landscape of human connection. It is an invitation to explore the various facets of intimacy, to understand the common obstacles that may impede its flourishing, and to discover strategies for nurturing and sustaining profound connections over time.

We will begin by examining the very essence of intimacy—what it means, how it manifests, and why it is integral to the human experience. From the intricacies of emotional connection to the nuances of physical touch, each chapter will unfold a layer of understanding, guiding you towards a richer comprehension of the multifaceted nature of intimacy.

Picture this book as a tapestry, and with each chapter, we will gently unveil a portion, revealing the intricacies and textures that make up the canvas of intimacy. From the delicate threads of communication to the bold strokes of passion, our journey is a deliberate unveiling—an exploration of the beauty and complexity woven into the fabric of deep connections.

As we traverse the terrain of intimacy, we will encounter obstacles that can obscure the path—communication breakdowns, unresolved conflicts, and the ebb and flow of desire. Fear not, for these challenges are not roadblocks but opportunities for growth, learning, and the strengthening of the bonds that tie us together.

This book serves as a guide, offering insights, practical tips, and reflective exercises to navigate the nuances of intimacy. Whether you are at the beginning of a relationship, seeking to reignite the flame in a longstanding connection, or simply curious about the intricacies of human connection, " Intimacy" is crafted to resonate with your journey.

So, let us embark on this voyage—one where the destination is not a fixed point but a continuous exploration of the richness and depth that intimacy can bring to your relationships. Let the unraveling of these pages guide you towards a more profound understanding of yourself and your connections with others. As we unveil the layers of intimacy, may you find inspiration, insights, and a renewed commitment to nurturing the connections that matter most. Welcome to a journey of discovery, growth, and the unwavering pursuit of deeper, more meaningful relationships.

DESIRE

Exploring the Depths of Desire:

Desire is the beating heart of intimacy, a complex interplay of emotions, thoughts, and physical sensations that form the essence of human connection. In this chapter, we delve into the psychology of desire, recognizing the nuances of individual differences and offering practical tips for communicating desires with a partner.

Recognizing Individual Variations:

Understanding desire requires an appreciation for the diverse ways in which individuals experience and express their sexual longing. We emphasize the importance of recognizing and respecting individual differences in sexual desire within a relationship, acknowledging that variations in intensity, frequency, and expression are natural aspects of human sexuality.

The Role of Emotions and Psychology:
Desire is profoundly influenced by emotional and psychological factors. We explore how past experiences, cultural influences, and personal beliefs shape the contours of desire, recognizing that a holistic understanding is crucial for fostering a supportive and empathetic connection.

The Interplay of Physical Sensations:
Physical sensations serve as the tangible expression of desire, bridging the gap between emotional longing and intimate connection. We delve into the interplay of physical sensations—arousal, touch, and sensory experiences—that contribute to the richness of desire, learning to attune to and appreciate the unique ways our bodies communicate and respond to desire.

Communicating Desires with a Partner:
Effective communication forms the bridge between individual desires and shared intimacy.

We offer practical tips for partners to communicate their desires openly and constructively, expressing needs and preferences, actively listening, and creating a safe space for vulnerability.

Creating a Language of Desire:
Desire often speaks in a language of its own, and partners can create a shared vocabulary that allows them to articulate and understand each other's longings. We explore the concept of creating a language of desire within a relationship—finding words, gestures, and cues that resonate with both partners—enhancing our ability to connect intimately and fulfill each other's desires.

Navigating Differences in Desire:
Differences in sexual desire are common within relationships, and navigating these variations requires sensitivity and communication. We provide insights into how partners can approach differences in desire, fostering a collaborative mindset that prioritizes understanding,

compromise, and the creation of a shared sexual narrative that accommodates the unique desires of both individuals.

SEX

Good sex is a highly personal and complex concept that involves a variety of physical, emotional, and psychological elements. It is important to note that what constitutes good sex can vary greatly between individuals, as everyone has different desires, boundaries, and expectations. Here are some key aspects often associated with the concept of good sex:

1. **Communication:** Open and honest communication is essential for good sex. Partners who talk about their wants, boundaries, and preferences are more likely to have a satisfying sexual experience. It is also important to actively listen to each other, making sure that both people feel heard and understood.

2. **Consent and Respect:** Good sex is consensual, with all parties involved willingly and enthusiastically participating. It is important to respect each other's boundaries, making sure

that everyone feels comfortable and safe throughout the encounter. Consent is an ongoing process that can be expressed verbally and non-verbally.

3. **Connection and Intimacy:** The emotional and intimate connection between partners is an important part of good sex. Feeling emotionally connected enhances the overall experience and contributes to a sense of closeness and vulnerability.

4. **Mutual Satisfaction:** Good sex is characterized by the satisfaction of all involved parties. This involves understanding each other's needs, preferences, and the ability to fulfill them. Partners should strive for mutual pleasure and make sure that each person's desires are taken into account.

5. **Variety and Exploration:** Variety and a willingness to explore different aspects of sexuality are important for good sex. This might include trying new activities, experimenting with

fantasies, and maintaining a sense of novelty to keep the sexual experience dynamic and exciting.

6. **Physical Enjoyment:** Physical pleasure is a major part of good sex. Partners should aim to understand each other's bodies, respond to cues of arousal, and prioritize each other's enjoyment. Paying attention to physical sensations, being responsive, and exploring erogenous zones can increase the pleasure of the experience.

7. **Embracing Individuality:** Recognizing and celebrating the uniqueness of each partner is essential for good sex. This involves appreciating individual desires, body types, and preferences without judgment, creating an environment of acceptance and self-expression.

Mindfulness and Presence in Sexual Intimacy

In the realm of sexual intimacy, mindfulness and presence can take a routine encounter and turn it into something truly special. By introducing mindfulness techniques, partners can become more aware of the present moment, savor it, and improve the quality of their sexual connection. Here, we look at the impact of being fully present and how practicing mindfulness can deepen connection and pleasure in intimate relationships.

1. **Introducing Mindfulness Techniques to Enhance the Present Moment:**

1.1 **Focused Breathing:**

Incorporating conscious and intentional breathing can help keep individuals in the present moment. Partners can sync their breath, creating a shared rhythm that encourages connection and increases awareness.

1.2 **Body Scan Meditation:**

A body scan meditation involves directing attention to different parts of the body, promoting a heightened sense of bodily awareness. Partners can take turns guiding each other through a body scan, deepening their connection to physical sensations.

1.3 **Sensory Awareness:**

Engaging the senses mindfully can improve the experience. Partners can explore touch, taste, smell, and sound deliberately, focusing on each sensation without distraction. This sensory awareness creates a richer and more immersive encounter.

1.4 **Mindful Movement:**

Incorporating slow and deliberate movements during intimate moments encourages mindfulness. Partners can explore the sensations of touch and movement with heightened awareness, creating a mindful dance that deepens their connection.

2. **The Impact of Being Fully Present on the Quality of the Experience:**

2.1 **Enhanced Sensitivity:**

Mindfulness amplifies sensitivity to physical and emotional cues. Being fully present allows partners to attune to each other's responses, fostering a deeper understanding of desires, preferences, and moments of heightened pleasure.

2.2 **Connection to Emotions:**

Presence in the moment enables a more profound connection to emotions. Partners can share vulnerability, express desires, and experience the full range of emotions together, deepening their emotional bond.

2.3 **Reduced Distractions:**

Mindfulness helps individuals let go of external distractions and mental chatter. By being fully present, partners create a space where external concerns fade away, allowing them to focus entirely on each other and the shared experience.

2.4 **Intensified Pleasure:**

The heightened awareness that comes with mindfulness can intensify physical pleasure. Partners can savor each sensation, creating a more profound and satisfying experience that goes beyond the physical act.

3. **Practicing Mindfulness to Deepen Connection and Pleasure:**

3.1 **Mindful Touch:**

Engaging in touch mindfully involves paying attention to the sensations and responses generated by each caress. Partners can explore the textures of each other's skin, fostering a deeper connection through touch.

3.2 **Eye Contact:**

Mindful eye contact establishes a profound connection between partners. Looking into each other's eyes with intentionality allows for a shared vulnerability and a sense of being truly seen and acknowledged.

3.3 **Shared Breathwork:**

Incorporating shared breathwork practices enhances connection. Partners can sync their breath, creating a shared rhythm that promotes unity and an intimate understanding of each other's internal states.

3.4 **Gratitude and Affirmations:**

Mindfulness extends beyond the physical to include emotional and relational aspects. Partners can express gratitude and affirmations mindfully, acknowledging each other's presence, contributions, and the shared journey of intimacy.

The Role of Foreplay in Intimate Connection

Foreplay is an essential part of sexual intimacy that is often overlooked. It involves a range of physical and emotional activities that help to increase arousal, create a connection, and lead to a more enjoyable sexual experience. Here, let's discuss the importance of foreplay, provide tips and techniques for engaging in intimate foreplay, and emphasize the need for mutual consent and communication during this important stage.

Foreplay is more than just a precursor to the main event—it is an integral part of the entire sexual experience. It serves several key purposes:

1. **Arousal and Excitement:**

Foreplay helps to build arousal and excitement, allowing both partners to transition from a state of relaxation to heightened sexual awareness.

This gradual buildup enhances sensitivity and anticipation.

2. **Emotional Connection:**

Engaging in foreplay fosters an emotional connection by creating an intimate space for partners to communicate, share desires, and express vulnerability. This emotional connection can deepen the overall satisfaction of the sexual encounter.

3. **Enhanced Physical Pleasure:**

By focusing on various erogenous zones and pleasure points, foreplay contributes to increased physical pleasure for both partners. This exploration sets the stage for a more fulfilling and satisfying sexual experience.

When it comes to engaging in intimate foreplay, communication is key. Expressing desires, preferences, and boundaries ensures that both partners feel comfortable and respected. Verbal and non-verbal cues play a crucial role in understanding each other's needs. Additionally, it is important to incorporate a variety of techniques and activities during foreplay, experiment with different types of touch, kisses, and caresses, and focus on erogenous zones. Sensory exploration can also be used to create a sensual atmosphere and heighten arousal. Introducing elements of teasing and anticipation can also intensify desire.

Mutual consent is essential at every stage of a sexual encounter, including foreplay. Both partners should feel comfortable expressing boundaries and have the autonomy to communicate their level of comfort throughout the process. Regularly check in with each other during foreplay to ensure that both partners are enjoying the experience and are comfortable with the activities.

Respect each other's boundaries without hesitation and create a safe and judgment-free space for open communication. Doing so will promote trust, understanding, and a shared sense of connection.

INTIMACY

In the complex web of human connection, intimacy is the vibrant thread that ties together the emotional, physical, and psychological aspects of relationships. It is more than just a fleeting moment of passion; it is the cornerstone of deep bonds, providing a profound understanding that goes beyond the surface. As we explore the significance of intimacy, we uncover the layers of its influence on the basis of relationships and the overall well-being of those involved.

Intimacy is not just about physical closeness; it is a powerful energy that breathes life into the spaces between partners, creating an atmosphere of trust, vulnerability, and shared experiences. It is the silent language of love, expressed through gestures, glances, and the gentle embrace of understanding.

In this journey, let us look into the various facets of intimacy, from the emotional connection that forms the foundation of relationships to the tangible expressions of physical closeness and the communication that bridges the gap between souls.

As we traverse the intricate landscape of human relationships, it becomes clear that intimacy is not a luxury but a fundamental requirement for the strong and lasting connection we seek. It is the force that unites two individuals into one, where acceptance, empathy, and shared aspirations form a bond that stands the test of time.

Join us on this exploration of the importance of intimacy, where we uncover its secrets, honor its beauty, and recognize its transformative power in forming relationships into havens of profound connection and unwavering love.

Emotional intimacy

In the vast expanse of human relationships, emotional intimacy is the foundation upon which strong connections are built. This chapter will take us on a journey into the realm of emotions, exploring the intricate threads that bind individuals together in a tapestry of profound understanding and closeness.

1.1 Grasping the Essence of Emotional Intimacy:

Emotional intimacy goes beyond the surface-level exchanges that often characterize casual interactions. It involves a deep exploration of one's inner world and an honest sharing of emotions with a partner. This section will delve into the essence of emotional intimacy, shedding light on its importance in creating a unique and irreplaceable bond.

1.2 The Power of Vulnerability:
Vulnerability is the key to emotional intimacy, inviting individuals to let down their guard and

reveal their true selves. This segment will examine the transformative power of vulnerability in relationships, highlighting its capacity to create an atmosphere where trust and authenticity can thrive.

1.3 Open Communication as the Cornerstone:
At the core of emotional intimacy lies the art of open communication. This section will explore the dynamics of sharing thoughts, feelings, and desires with a partner in a transparent and non-judgmental space. It will unravel the importance of effective communication as the building block for emotional intimacy, fostering an environment where mutual understanding can flourish.

1.4 Strengthening Trust Through Emotional Intimacy:
Trust, a delicate yet powerful element, is closely linked to emotional intimacy. This segment will delve into the symbiotic relationship between trust and emotional closeness, elucidating how the vulnerability shared in intimate moments

contributes to the strengthening of trust. Trust becomes the glue that binds partners together, creating a solid foundation for a lasting connection.

1.5 Understanding and Empathy:
Emotional intimacy cultivates a deep sense of understanding and empathy between partners. This section will examine the role of empathy in fostering emotional connection, emphasizing the importance of actively listening and attuning to a partner's emotional landscape. Through shared experiences and empathetic gestures, partners develop a profound understanding that fortifies the emotional bond.

1.6 The Profound Sense of Connection:
Emotional intimacy, at its peak, results in a profound and unspoken connection between partners. This segment will explore the nuanced ways in which emotional closeness manifests, transcending the boundaries of language and reaching into the realm of shared emotions. It will paint a picture of a relationship where

partners feel not just heard but truly seen, understood, and valued.

Physical Intimacy

Physical closeness, a dance of touch and nearness, adds a dynamic layer to the complex texture of human connection. In this chapter, we investigate the importance of physical contact, the biochemical responses that underlie it, and the fundamental job it plays in keeping up a flourishing and sound relationship.

2.1 The Language of Touch:

Physical contact fills in as a powerful and all-inclusive language of association. This segment investigates the different manners by which touch communicates love, fondness, and comprehension between accomplices. From the unobtrusive brush of fingertips to the warmth of an embrace, physical closeness sets up a material extension between people.

2.2 Oxytocin, the "Love Hormone":

At the physiological center of physical closeness lies oxytocin, regularly alluded to as the "love hormone." This area unravels the intricate biochemical procedures activated by physical contact, investigating how oxytocin advances bonding, trust, and passionate association between accomplices. Comprehending the job of this hormone gives understanding into the extraordinary effect of physical closeness on the passionate scene of a relationship.

2.3 The Power of Bonding:

Physical closeness fills in as a trigger for bonding, making a one of a kind shared encounter between accomplices. This area examines how shared snapshots of physical closeness add to a feeling of solidarity and togetherness. It features the transformative intensity of physical association in deepening the passionate bond, encouraging a feeling of security and having a place.

2.4 The Spectrum of Physical Intimacy:

Past the domain of sexual experiences, physical closeness covers a range of encounters. This piece of the chapter investigates the different articulations of physical nearness, including cuddling, holding hands, and non-sexual contact. Acknowledging the various manners by which accomplices can associate physically upgrades the wealth and adaptability of the physical measurement inside a relationship.

2.5 Sexual Satisfaction and Relationship Health:

While physical closeness reaches out past sexual experiences, sexual fulfillment stays a basic part of a sound relationship. This area talks about the job of sexual fulfillment in keeping up a strong and fulfilling association. It investigates the mutuality between passionate and physical closeness, accentuating the significance of a fulfilling sexual relationship in advancing general relationship prosperity.

2.6 Navigating Challenges in Physical Intimacy:

Physical closeness may experience difficulties, running from contrasts in craving to outside stressors affecting the close association between accomplices. This area gives understanding into exploring these difficulties with open correspondence, sympathy, and a shared responsibility to keeping up a sound physical association.

Spiritual intimacy

Amidst the realms of emotional and physical connection, the ethereal dimension of spiritual intimacy emerges as a powerful force in forming the basis of profound and long-lasting relationships. In this chapter, we will explore the importance of shared values, beliefs, and life goals, and how a sense of spiritual connection can contribute to the richness and longevity of a meaningful relationship.

At the core of spiritual intimacy lies the recognition and alignment of shared values and beliefs. It is essential to identify common ground in matters of ethics, morality, and worldview. When partners find resonance in their fundamental principles, a strong spiritual foundation begins to form, providing a compass that guides the relationship through life's many experiences.

Spiritual intimacy fosters a sense of unity and connection that goes beyond the tangible world.

This segment looks into the transcendental aspects of shared spiritual values, emphasizing how they create a deeper, more profound connection between partners. As the relationship is infused with shared meaning, it evolves into a shared spiritual journey.

Spiritual intimacy often finds expression in meaningful rituals and traditions shared between partners. This part of the chapter examines the role of these practices in solidifying a sense of unity and continuity. Whether through shared ceremonies, celebrations, or daily rituals, these activities contribute to the creation of a sacred space within the relationship.

A shared sense of purpose acts as a driving force that propels the relationship forward. This section explores how spiritual intimacy gives rise to a collective vision, inspiring partners to pursue shared goals and aspirations. As each individual's journey aligns with the overarching purpose of the relationship, a harmonious and fulfilling dynamic emerges.

Spiritual intimacy serves as a catalyst for personal and collective growth. This part of the chapter delves into how shared spiritual values encourage continuous self-discovery and evolution. By supporting each other's individual growth and transformation, partners contribute to the overall development of the relationship, creating a synergy that transcends the mundane and enriches the shared journey.

Even in the realm of spiritual intimacy, challenges may arise. This segment looks into how a shared spiritual connection provides a source of strength and resilience during difficult times. The common ground in beliefs and values acts as a stabilizing force, helping partners navigate challenges with a shared understanding and commitment to overcoming adversity.

Intellectual Intimacy

Amidst the vast array of human connection, intellectual intimacy stands out as a beacon, highlighting the profound bond that can be formed through mental connection and shared interests. In this chapter, we will delve into the realms of cognition and curiosity, exploring the transformative power of intellectual engagement and its essential role in creating a unique and lasting connection.

4.1 The Significance of Mental Connection:

Intellectual intimacy emphasizes the importance of mental connection between partners. This section will shed light on the depth that shared intellectual interests bring to a relationship, forming a special kind of intimacy that goes beyond the physical. By aligning cognitive wavelengths, partners embark on a journey of mutual exploration and understanding.

4.2 Encouraging Intellectual Pursuits:

The path to intellectual intimacy is paved with stimulating conversations, shared discoveries, and a commitment to ongoing learning. This part of the chapter encourages partners to actively engage in intellectual activities, whether through shared hobbies, educational endeavors, or simply exchanging ideas on topics of mutual interest. Intellectual engagement becomes a dynamic force, bringing life to the relationship.

4.3 The Art of Stimulating Discussions:

At the core of intellectual intimacy lies the art of conversation. This section will explore the nuances of stimulating dialogues—conversations that challenge, inspire, and spark curiosity. Partners learn to appreciate the exchange of ideas, cultivating an environment where intellectual growth is not only encouraged but celebrated as an integral part of the relationship.

4.4 Curiosity as a Driving Force:

Curiosity becomes the catalyst for intellectual exploration within a relationship. This segment will delve into the role of curiosity as a driving force, inspiring partners to seek knowledge, ask questions, and embark on shared intellectual adventures. Nurturing a sense of wonder and inquisitiveness becomes the cornerstone for a thriving intellectual connection.

4.5 Shared Interests as a Bonding Agent:

Common interests serve as a powerful bonding agent, weaving partners into a shared narrative of exploration and discovery. This part of the chapter will explore the various ways in which shared hobbies, passions, or pursuits contribute to intellectual intimacy. As partners collaborate in their pursuits, a unique intellectual synergy emerges, strengthening the fabric of the relationship.

4.6 Mutual Respect in Intellectual Intimacy:

The foundation of intellectual intimacy rests on a bedrock of mutual respect. This section will emphasize the importance of respecting each other's thoughts, opinions, and perspectives. Intellectual disagreements are approached with an understanding that diversity of thought enriches the relationship, fostering an environment where differing viewpoints are valued and appreciated.

Recreational Intimacy

In the kaleidoscope of human connection, recreational intimacy is a vivid palette, adding color to the canvas of shared experiences. This chapter encourages us to explore the joy and connection that can be found when partners engage in activities together, create common hobbies, and enjoy the lightness of laughter and playfulness.

Quality time is the currency of love, and this section looks into the profound advantages of spending meaningful moments together. Whether it's leisurely pursuits or thrilling adventures, the time shared becomes the foundation for making memories and deepening the connection between partners. Recreational intimacy turns ordinary moments into extraordinary bonds.

Shared hobbies and experiences are the foundation of recreational intimacy. This part of the chapter examines the many possibilities for partners to find common interests and pursuits. Whether it's trying out new cuisines, delving into artistic endeavors, or embarking on outdoor adventures, creating shared experiences can be a source of joy and connection within the relationship.

Laughter, the universal language of joy, is a key part of recreational intimacy. This section highlights the transformative power of shared laughter, examining how humor can dissolve tension, create moments of genuine connection, and act as a bridge between partners. In the tapestry of a relationship, laughter stitches together the fabric of shared joy.

Playfulness brings an element of spontaneity and light-heartedness into a relationship. This segment looks at the role of playfulness in recreational intimacy, encouraging partners to engage in activities that bring joy, foster creativity, and break away from the routine. Through playfulness, partners can discover new sides of each other and cultivate a sense of adventure within the relationship.

Discovering and navigating shared interests requires openness and a spirit of exploration. This part of the chapter provides insights into how partners can identify common hobbies that resonate with both, fostering a sense of togetherness. From the simple pleasures of a shared book club to the excitement of pursuing a mutual passion, shared interests become the threads that weave the fabric of recreational intimacy.

Recreational intimacy is a conduit for building connection, and this section looks at how playfulness contributes to this dynamic. Engaging in activities that involve shared goals, friendly competition, or collaborative problem-solving can enhance the sense of teamwork and camaraderie. As partners play together, they can strengthen their bond and create lasting memories.

Cultivating Intimacy Over Time in Long-Term Relationships

Maintaining intimacy in long-term relationships is a rewarding endeavor that requires effort and intentionality. To keep the connection alive, it's important to employ strategies, be adaptable, and celebrate milestones. Here, we discuss effective tactics for sustaining intimacy, the importance of growth and adaptability, and the significance of creating new shared experiences.

When it comes to strategies for keeping intimacy alive, prioritize quality time. Dedicate time to each other that goes beyond daily routines and responsibilities. Schedule date nights, engage in activities you both enjoy, and have meaningful conversations to deepen your connection. Additionally, maintain open and honest communication. Check in with each other about your feelings, desires, and the state of your relationship. Create a safe space for vulnerability, ensuring that both partners feel heard and understood.

In addition to strategies, it's important to embrace change and support individual development. Recognize that both individuals and relationships evolve over time and view these changes as opportunities for growth. Encourage each other's personal growth and development, and revisit and reaffirm shared goals and values. When life throws challenges your way, embrace them as opportunities for mutual support, problem-solving, and reinforcing the resilience of your relationship.

Finally, celebrate milestones and create new traditions. Mark important occasions that hold significance for your relationship, such as anniversaries or major life events. Establish new traditions as your relationship evolves, such as annual getaways or special rituals. Embark on new adventures together, and express gratitude for each other and the journey you've shared. Celebrate the small moments and achievements, reinforcing the positive aspects of your relationship and fostering a culture of appreciation.

Building Trust And Security

In relationships, trust is the key element that keeps the balance between vulnerability and connection. This chapter looks into the relationship between trust and intimacy, and provides strategies for creating and sustaining trust, as well as the positive effect of a secure emotional base on all aspects of a relationship.

6.1 Trust and Intimacy:

Trust is the foundation on which intimacy is built. This section examines the relationship between trust and intimacy, and how the ability to rely on a partner encourages a deeper level of vulnerability, openness, and connection. Trust is the currency that allows for emotional and physical closeness.

6.2 Building Trust:

Constructing trust is a conscious effort. This part of the chapter outlines practical methods for nurturing trust in a relationship. From open communication and transparency to dependability and consistency, partners discover the components that contribute to a strong foundation of trust. Establishing trust is an ongoing process that requires dedication and mutual understanding.

6.3 Honesty and Transparency:

At the core of trust is the promise of honesty and transparency. This section looks into the role of open communication in creating an atmosphere where partners feel safe to share their thoughts, feelings, and vulnerabilities. Honest conversations are the crucible in which trust is formed, leading to emotional intimacy that permeates the relationship.

6.4 Reliability and Consistency:

Reliability and consistency are the pillars of trust, providing partners with a sense of security and predictability. This part of the chapter delves into the importance of being dependable and maintaining consistency in actions and behaviors. Through reliability, partners create a sense of safety that serves as the scaffolding for a trusting relationship.

6.5 Forgiveness and Repair:

Acknowledging that trust may be challenged, this part of the chapter looks into the roles of forgiveness and repair in restoring trust. Partners learn to manage conflicts with empathy and a commitment to understanding, creating an environment where mistakes become chances for growth and the rebuilding of trust.

6.6 The Impact of a Secure Emotional Foundation:

A secure emotional foundation is the fertile soil in which trust and intimacy can thrive. This section highlights the profound effect of emotional security on all aspects of a relationship. Partners who feel emotionally secure are more likely to engage in open communication, express vulnerability, and explore various dimensions of intimacy with confidence.

6.7 Vulnerability as a Bridge to Trust: Vulnerability is the bridge that links trust and intimacy. This segment examines how partners can navigate the delicate dance of vulnerability, gradually revealing parts of themselves to one another. In the safety of trust, vulnerability becomes a catalyst for deeper emotional connection and a more meaningful intimacy.

INTIMACY BEYOND THE BEDROOM

As we move beyond the bedroom, a world of non-sexual intimacy opens up, inviting us to explore the deep connection that can be created in the everyday. This chapter looks at the various forms of intimacy that don't involve sex, celebrating the power of small gestures, shared moments, and the art of expressing love in meaningful ways.

7.1 Non-Sexual Forms of Intimacy:

Intimacy comes in many forms, and it doesn't always have to be sexual. This section looks at the different types of non-sexual intimacy, from the warmth of a gentle touch to the comfort of shared silences. Partners can learn to connect on a deeply personal level without the need for sex.

7.2 Cuddling, Holding Hands, and Intimate Gestures:

Non-sexual touch can be its own language, expressing love and connection in both subtle and profound ways. This part of the chapter looks at the importance of cuddling, holding hands, and other intimate gestures that can't be put into words. Partners can learn to communicate affection and closeness through touch, creating a language that's unique to their relationship.

7.3 Small, Everyday Moments:

The fabric of intimacy is made up of small, everyday moments. This section looks at the impact of seemingly mundane interactions—the shared glances, smiles, and fleeting touches that add up to a strong connection. Partners can find intimacy in the simplicity of daily life, not just in grand gestures.

7.4 Building a Sense of Togetherness:

A sense of togetherness is built through intentional presence and shared experiences. This segment looks at the importance of being present in each other's lives, participating in the everyday rituals that create a feeling of unity. Partners can discover that true togetherness is made up of small, consistent moments, not just big events.

7.5 Expressing Love in Various Ways:

The expression of love goes beyond the romantic, extending into all aspects of life. This part of the chapter encourages partners to find unique and personal ways to express affection. From thoughtful gestures to acts of service, partners can learn to communicate love in ways that fit the individual dynamics of their relationship.

7.6 Shared Projects and Collaborations:

Collaborative endeavors can be a way to create non-sexual intimacy, fostering a sense of partnership and shared purpose. This section looks at the importance of embarking on shared projects or pursuing mutual interests, allowing partners to engage in activities that deepen their connection and create lasting memories beyond the bedroom.

7.7 Celebrating Each Other's Individuality:

Non-sexual intimacy involves celebrating each other's individuality and appreciating the unique qualities that make each partner who they are. This segment encourages partners to express love by acknowledging and supporting each other's personal growth, aspirations, and individual passions.

Creating A Comfortable Space For Intimacy

Creating a comfortable and secure physical environment is essential for fostering intimacy in a relationship. The bedroom, in particular, is a significant factor in shaping the overall experience. Here, we'll discuss the importance of a comfortable setting and provide tips for designing a bedroom that encourages intimacy through thoughtful considerations of lighting, decor, and ambiance.

A comfortable space is key for allowing vulnerability, trust, and emotional connection. When individuals feel safe and at ease in their environment, they are more likely to open up and share intimate moments with their partner. A comfortable space is not just physical; it also extends to the emotional safety created by mutual respect and understanding.

When it comes to designing a bedroom conducive to intimacy, lighting is a crucial factor. Soft, dimmable lighting can contribute to a more relaxed and intimate atmosphere. Consider using bedside lamps, string lights, or candles to create a warm and inviting glow. Avoid harsh, bright lights that may feel clinical or sterile.

Decor should reflect the personal tastes and preferences of both partners. Keep the space clutter-free and opt for soothing colors that promote relaxation. Personal touches, such as meaningful artwork or sentimental items, can add a sense of connection and familiarity.

Ambiance is the overall mood or atmosphere of the space. Consider incorporating elements that enhance the romantic feel of the bedroom. Soft fabrics, comfortable bedding, and sensual textures can contribute to a cozy and inviting atmosphere. Experiment with scents, such as calming essential oils or candles, to add an olfactory dimension to the ambiance.

Invest in comfortable and inviting furniture that encourages relaxation. A well-chosen mattress, plush pillows, and soft linens can significantly enhance the comfort of the bedroom. Ensure that the furniture arrangement promotes easy movement and accessibility for both partners.

Maintaining a comfortable temperature is crucial for creating a cozy environment. Be mindful of the room's temperature and provide options for regulating warmth, such as extra blankets or a fan. Striking the right balance ensures that both partners feel physically comfortable and can fully enjoy the intimate experience.

Infuse the space with elements that hold personal significance for both partners. This might include photographs, mementos, or items that evoke shared memories. Creating a bedroom that reflects the unique identity of the relationship enhances the sense of intimacy and connection.

Establishing a sense of privacy and security is essential for intimacy. Consider window treatments that provide adequate privacy and minimize outside disturbances. Ensure that the bedroom door can be securely closed, allowing partners to focus on each other without external interruptions.

Make the bedroom a technology-free zone to minimize distractions. The absence of electronic devices promotes focused attention on each other, allowing for deeper emotional connection and intimacy.

Spicing Things UP

As relationships develop, it's natural to want to add some excitement and variety to the bedroom. This chapter looks at how partners can do this, from trying new positions and activities to exploring fantasies and sensory pleasures. It's important to create a safe and non-judgmental space where partners can openly communicate their desires and preferences.

Playfulness and creativity can also be incorporated to break away from routine and add a sense of joy and spontaneity. Ultimately, the goal is to prioritize mutual satisfaction and pleasure, creating a shared space of enjoyment that enhances the intimate connection.

BODY POSITIVITY AND Self Love

In the intricate dance of intimacy, the way we feel about our bodies has a huge impact on our self-esteem and sexual confidence. This chapter looks at the journey of embracing body positivity, nurturing self-love, and creating an atmosphere that encourages a positive body image in both partners.

9.1 Embracing Body Positivity:

Body positivity is all about celebrating the different shapes, sizes, and forms that make us unique. This section looks at the importance of embracing body positivity as a way to build a healthier self-image. Partners can appreciate the beauty in their own bodies and appreciate the uniqueness of each other, creating an environment where self-love can grow.

9.2 The Impact of Self-Love on Sexual Confidence:

Self-love is the key to sexual confidence, influencing how we feel about ourselves in intimate moments. This part of the chapter looks at the power of cultivating self-love, and how having a positive self-image can lead to increased sexual confidence. Partners learn that by embracing and cherishing their own bodies, they can be more secure and empowered in the bedroom.

9.3 Nurturing Self-Love:

Nurturing self-love is an ongoing process that requires self-compassion and acceptance. This section provides practical strategies for cultivating self-love, from positive affirmations to self-care and activities that promote a positive body image. Partners can go on a journey of self-discovery and self-acceptance, learning to love themselves in a holistic way.

9.4 Encouraging Positive Body Image in Your Partner:

Creating a supportive environment for positive body image is not just about ourselves, but also about our relationship. This segment looks at how partners can actively contribute to each other's body positivity. Partners can learn to give genuine compliments, create a safe space for vulnerability, and celebrate each other's bodies, creating an atmosphere where both individuals feel seen and appreciated.

9.5 Challenging Societal Beauty Standards:

Societal beauty standards can create unrealistic expectations, affecting our perceptions of our bodies. This part of the chapter encourages partners to challenge and redefine these standards within the context of their relationship. By celebrating the authenticity of each other's bodies, couples can reject harmful narratives and create a space that values genuine beauty and self-acceptance.

9.6 Intimacy as a Journey of Connection:

Embracing body positivity and self-love changes the journey of intimacy into a shared exploration of connection. This section emphasizes that intimacy is not about conforming to external ideals but about creating a space where partners can express vulnerability, celebrate uniqueness, and experience the profound connection that comes from embracing each other's bodies with love and acceptance.

9.7 Sustaining Body Positivity in the Relationship:

Sustaining body positivity is an ongoing commitment within a relationship. This segment looks at how partners can continue to prioritize and reinforce body positivity as they navigate life together. By creating an atmosphere of unconditional acceptance and genuine admiration for each other's bodies, couples can build a strong foundation for a healthy and fulfilling intimate connection.

Technology And Intimacy

In the digital age, technology has become an integral part of modern relationships, influencing how couples interact and share intimate moments. This chapter looks at the multifaceted role of technology in intimacy, discussing its potential advantages, ways to strengthen the bond, and the importance of setting healthy boundaries for technology use in the relationship.

10.1 Exploring the Role of Technology in Modern Relationships:

Technology has become a part of our everyday lives, impacting how we communicate and connect. This section examines the ever-changing role of technology in modern relationships, analyzing how digital tools shape the dynamics of intimacy. Couples can recognize the positive aspects of technology, such as its ability to bridge distances, facilitate communication, and enhance shared experiences.

10.2 Leveraging Technology for Enhanced Intimacy:

Although technology can present challenges, it also offers unique opportunities to increase intimacy. This part of the chapter looks at how couples can use technology to foster connection and deepen their bond. From virtual date nights to shared playlists and intimate messages, partners can discover creative ways to use technology as a tool for enriching their relationship.

10.3 The Impact of Social Media on Intimacy:

Social media plays a major role in how couples share their lives with the world. This section examines the impact of social media on intimacy, exploring the balance between sharing moments with a wider audience and preserving private, intimate spaces within the relationship.

Partners can learn to navigate the digital landscape mindfully, protecting the sanctity of their shared experiences.

10.4 Intimacy in the Age of Video Calls: Video calls have become a lifeline for keeping in touch in long-distance relationships. This segment looks at how couples can use video calls to create a sense of presence and closeness, despite physical distances. Partners can appreciate the nuances of virtual connection, recognizing the potential for meaningful moments even through a screen.

10.5 Setting Healthy Boundaries for Technology Use:
As technology infiltrates intimate spaces, setting healthy boundaries is essential. This part of the chapter provides guidance on establishing clear and respectful limits on technology use within the relationship. Couples can explore the importance of being present in the moment, creating quality time without distractions, and

designating tech-free spaces, especially in the bedroom.

10.6 Mindful Communication in the Digital Age:
Effective communication is key to intimate connections, even in the digital age. This section looks at the nuances of mindful communication in the context of technology, emphasizing the importance of active listening, expressing needs and desires, and maintaining open dialogue. Couples can discover how intentional communication can foster deeper understanding and connection.

10.7 Balancing Digital and Physical Intimacy:
Although technology can enhance certain aspects of intimacy, it's important to balance digital connections with physical presence. This segment examines how couples can navigate the delicate balance between digital and physical intimacy, making sure that the appeal of screens doesn't overshadow the richness of face-to-face interactions.

Exploring Fantasies

11.1 Understanding the Role of Fantasies in a Healthy Sex Life:

Fantasies can be a powerful tool to add a layer of excitement and exploration to a healthy sex life. This chapter looks into the importance of fantasies, providing insight into how to communicate and experiment with them, as well as the need for trust and safety when exploring new experiences.

11.2 Communicating Fantasies:

Sharing fantasies requires open and non-judgmental communication. This part of the chapter emphasizes the importance of creating a safe space for partners to express their desires and fantasies. Couples can learn how to communicate effectively, making sure that the sharing of fantasies is met with understanding, respect, and a shared commitment to mutual exploration.

11.3 Experimenting with Fantasies:

Fantasies offer a great opportunity for experimentation, allowing couples to explore new dimensions of intimacy together. This section looks into the process of experimenting with fantasies, encouraging partners to approach these experiences with curiosity and a willingness to learn. Partners can learn how to navigate the realms of role-playing, sensory exploration, and other fantasy-driven activities that can enhance their sexual connection.

11.4 Establishing Trust and Safety:

Trust and safety are essential when exploring fantasies. This segment explores the importance of establishing a foundation of trust between partners, making sure that both individuals feel secure and respected in their vulnerabilities. Partners can discover that trust creates a container within which fantasies can be freely expressed and explored without fear of judgment.

11.5 Building a Shared Fantasy Space:

As couples embark on the journey of exploring fantasies, they can build a shared fantasy space—a realm that is co-created and maintained by both partners. This part of the chapter provides insight into fostering an environment where mutual fantasies are respected, and boundaries are clearly communicated. Partners can learn how to create a space where experimentation is celebrated and the exploration of desires becomes a shared adventure.

11.6 Embracing Individual and Shared Fantasies:

Fantasies can be both individual and shared, adding depth and diversity to a couple's sexual repertoire. This section looks into the beauty of embracing both personal and mutual fantasies, recognizing that the interplay between individual desires and shared exploration contributes to a dynamic and fulfilling sexual connection.

11.7 Post-Exploration Reflection and Communication:

After the exploration of fantasies, reflection and communication become crucial components of the journey. This segment guides partners in discussing their experiences, expressing feelings, and learning from the shared exploration. Effective post-exploration communication can help foster continued understanding, trust, and connection within the relationship.

The Art Of Seduction

Seduction is an art that weaves together excitement, mystery, and passion to create intimate connections. This chapter looks at the nuances of seduction, offering advice on how to rekindle the thrill of new beginnings, keep the spark alive in long-term relationships, and express desire in creative ways.

Rediscovering the Excitement of Seduction:

It is possible to rekindle the excitement of seduction even in a long-term relationship. This section looks at how to bring spontaneity, playfulness, and anticipation into your intimate interactions, breathing new life into the art of seduction.

Tips for Keeping the Spark Alive in Long-Term Relationships:

Long-term relationships need to be nurtured to keep the flame of desire alive. This part of the chapter provides practical tips on how to do this, such as cultivating curiosity and exploration, embracing novelty and surprise, celebrating milestones, and creating shared fantasies.

Creating a Sensual Environment:

The atmosphere in which seduction takes place is key to its allure. This section looks at how to craft an environment that invites intimacy and intensifies the art of seduction, from setting the mood with lighting, music, and scents to incorporating tactile elements.

Embracing Spontaneity and Playfulness:

Seduction is enhanced by spontaneity and playfulness. This segment encourages partners to embrace the element of surprise, introducing unexpected moments of connection and delight. Couples learn to infuse playfulness into their interactions, making the ordinary extraordinary.

Expressing Desire Through Words and Gestures:

Verbal and non-verbal communication can be powerful tools in the art of seduction. This part of the chapter explores how to express desire through words and gestures, such as articulating longings, offering compliments, and using body language to convey passion and attraction.

Incorporating Fantasy and Role-Playing:

Fantasy and role-playing can add excitement and novelty to the art of seduction. This section guides partners in exploring creative scenarios, sharing fantasies, and engaging in role-playing activities that tap into the realms of imagination.

Sustaining Passionate Connection:

Passionate connection is sustained when partners prioritize and invest in the ongoing art of seduction. This segment emphasizes the importance of making time for each other, maintaining open communication about desires, and actively participating in the dance of seduction.

Sustaining a Fulfilling Sex Life

As relationships progress, it takes intention, communication, and a commitment to ongoing growth to keep a fulfilling sex life. This last chapter looks at strategies for long-term satisfaction, emphasizing the need for continuous communication and recognizing the ever-changing nature of the relationship to ensure a dynamic and enjoyable sexual connection.

12.1 Strategies for Long-Term Satisfaction:

Having a fulfilling sex life over the long haul requires a strategic and thoughtful approach. This section looks at practical strategies for long-term satisfaction, from making intimacy a priority in the relationship to exploring new activities and keeping things fresh. Partners learn to adjust to the changing dynamics of their relationship, understanding that sustaining fulfillment takes effort, creativity, and a willingness to explore together.

12.2 Prioritizing Intimacy in the Relationship:

Intimacy is essential for a fulfilling sex life, and making it a priority in the relationship is key. This part of the chapter looks at how couples can make intentional efforts to foster intimacy in various aspects of their lives. From emotional connection to shared experiences and physical closeness, partners learn to weave intimacy into the fabric of their relationship.

12.3 Embracing the Evolving Nature of Desire:

Desire is ever-changing, and acknowledging its evolving nature is essential for long-term satisfaction. This section helps partners accept the changes in desires and preferences that may occur over time. By staying attuned to each other's needs and communicating openly about evolving desires, couples can navigate the ever-changing landscape of their sexual connection.

12.4 Experimentation and Novelty:

Experimentation and novelty bring vitality to a long-term sexual relationship. This segment looks at the importance of trying new activities, exploring fantasies, and introducing variety into the intimate aspects of the relationship. Partners learn to approach experimentation with curiosity, creating an atmosphere where ongoing exploration is valued and encouraged.

12.5 Continuous Communication:

Open and continuous communication is the lifeblood of a fulfilling sex life. This part of the chapter emphasizes the importance of maintaining a dialogue about desires, boundaries, and the overall satisfaction within the relationship. Partners learn to express their needs and actively listen to each other, creating an environment where communication fosters understanding and connection.

12.6 Cultivating Emotional Connection:

Emotional connection serves as the foundation for a deeply satisfying sex life. This section looks at how partners can cultivate and nurture emotional intimacy, recognizing that the emotional bond between them directly influences the quality of their sexual connection. Strategies for deepening emotional connection include shared vulnerability, mutual support, and active engagement in each other's lives.

12.7 Prioritizing Relationship Growth:

As the relationship evolves, prioritizing ongoing growth is essential for sustaining a fulfilling sex life. This segment encourages partners to view the relationship as a dynamic journey, embracing opportunities for individual and collective growth. By fostering an environment that encourages continuous learning, exploration, and personal development, couples create a foundation for a fulfilling and evolving connection.

CONCLUSION

As we come to the end of our exploration of intimacy, let us take a moment to reflect on the incredible journey we have taken together. We have delved into the complexities of human connection, vulnerability, and the delicate art of intimacy. "Intimacy: Nurturing Deeper Connections in Relationships" has been our guide, helping us to navigate the maze of emotions, desires, and shared experiences that make up the fabric of our relationships.

Think of the relationships in your life as a vibrant and ever-changing tapestry, made up of joy, struggles, laughter, and sometimes tears. This book has sought to unravel the intricacies of that tapestry, allowing you to examine each thread, each knot, and each color that contributes to the unique beauty of your connections.

We have learned that intimacy is not a perfect work of art, but a living, breathing creation that grows and adapts over time. It is in the imperfections, the raw and unfiltered moments, that the true beauty of intimacy is revealed. It is in these imperfections that we find the authenticity and depth that make our connections truly meaningful.

Our journey has not been about reaching a destination, but about understanding that intimacy is an ongoing process of growth and exploration. Every relationship is a work in progress, a canvas waiting for new strokes, new patterns, and the ever-evolving story of connection.

Remember that the power to cultivate intimacy lies in the choices you make every day. The choice to communicate openly, the choice to be vulnerable, and the choice to actively nurture the bonds that matter. These seemingly small choices can have a huge impact on the quality and depth of your relationships.

Intimacy flourishes in the soil of vulnerability. It is in the moments when we allow ourselves to be seen—the unfiltered, unedited version—that intimacy blooms. Embrace vulnerability as a source of strength, a bridge for deeper understanding, and a catalyst for profound connections.

As we come to a close, keep in mind that nurturing intimacy is a lifelong commitment—an ongoing dance that requires attentiveness, adaptability, and a genuine investment in the well-being of your relationships.

This book is not the end, but a stepping stone, a guide that encourages you to continue the journey of exploration and growth. Take the insights, strategies, and lessons you have learned and apply them to your everyday interactions.

As you embark on your own intimate journey, may you find fulfillment, joy, and a renewed appreciation for the ever-evolving tapestry of human connection. May the understanding you have gained here stay with you as a reminder of the potential within your relationships—the potential for deeper connections, shared vulnerability, and the enduring beauty of intimacy.

The End

www.ingramcontent.com/pod-product-compliance
Lightning Source LLC
Chambersburg PA
CBHW070752250726
48662CB00004B/1764